KAMASUTRA

SEX POSITIONS

GUIDE

The ultimate Kama sutra guide, tantric sex positions that will transform your sexual life. Techniques for incredible lovemaking. Increase intimacy in your relationships.

Sarah Streep

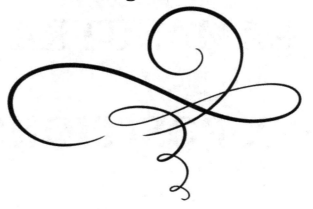

Table of contents

5

Introduction

Throughout this book, you will discover the history of Kama Sutra, the beliefs and practices surrounding it, the practice itself, and how it relates to modern-day sexual desires and fantasies, as well as how you can bring the Kama Sutra into your bedroom. As an activity that we all engage in, sex can be as intimate or as artificial as your desire. As times continue, sex has become more of a casual encounter among lustful individuals than a passionate lovemaking activity. We've laid this book out to be able to teach you the ways of the Kama Sutra so you can bring passionate lovemaking into your bedroom.

The Kama Sutra takes you back to the origin of lovemaking at its finest, and somewhat uncanny practices, to help you discover yourself, your significant other, and what pleasure means to you and your relationship. Kama Sutra will teach you how to find joy in pleasuring someone else, and how to find pleasure through a series of locations on the body that are easily overlooked, especially during foreplay.

This book provides an overview of the most popular practices and techniques surrounding Kama Sutra. Though many may disagree with certain aspects and beliefs surrounding Kama Sutra, it is intended only to educate one on the matters, not to convert you. Even if you decide that you do not agree with the beliefs around the Kama Sutra, you are sure to take something beneficial away from the book, alsoif it is just a new foreplay technique or poses you want to try with a lover. Although based on Hindu beliefs, people from all walks of life and all religions, to attain pleasure during foreplay, sexual intercourse, marriage, and relationships, can practice Kama Sutra.

This book will give you insight into the practices of Kama Sutra, what is expected from a couple in the relationship, and the bedroom. This book will also make you aware of the general guidelines which male and females follow when attempting to pursue one another. There is also a general overview of what practices are allowed or permitted after the wedding day. It is an exciting topic that is worthy of exploring more about, and I hope you will be able to put some things into practice.

Sex is an essential part of a romantic relationship for many reasons. While it is noted to have a variety of excellent health benefits (such as stimulating happiness, easing depression, headaches, and other ailments), it is also an essential part of developing the bond between you and your partner. Having sex with your partner helps increase the amount of intimacy, romance, and trust that you experience in your relationship. It encourages both partners to feel close in a way that they don't share with anyone else. There are many reasons why sex is healthy in a relationship.

As you read this book, you will discover a variety of phenomenal advice for couples. From how to turn each other on, to different moves, and toys to try, there is something in store for every couple. This book is intended for any intensity of lovers, from modest to downright crazy, and even a special section for anal. You can be sure that you will find something that is going to please both you and your partner.

This book is geared towards couples and has advice on moves and techniques that can enhance the intimacy and deepen the romance between lovers. Every single stepor tip in this book will either assist in developing the intimate bonds between you two or encourage you to have total trust in your partner while you are in a vulnerable state. Some moves are slow and relaxed, ones that will have you and your partner in a steamy face to face position and ones that will allow for you to let your wild side take over. Whichever you choose, you are guaranteed to make sparks fly and drive each other to unforgettable orgasms.

It is important to read this book together as a couple, as it can help encourage an open line of communication in the bedroom. This area of discussion is just as important as elsewhere, as it helps us convey what we want and what we don't want. Many people don't realize that we tend to evolve in our sexual desires the same way as we developand grow elsewhere in life. Because of this, we may have different fetishes, curiosities, or desires as we grow. By communicating with your partner, you can help teach them how to pleasure you in the way you want.

Additionally, you should be sure that the communication includes discussing what you *don't* want or like. These things should be made very clear, and there should be no pressure on the denying party to change their minds. The key is to keep the trust and respect strong between the two of you, so the two of you can further enhance the romance and intimacy. If the other is not on board with something, do not pressure them to feel the need to be. Should they change their mind down the road, let them come to you: do not under any circumstances pressure or force your partner to engage in romance they don't want.

Through open lines of communication, you may discover new or unspoken desires that your spouse may have. These conversations are great, as they encourage you to try new things and bring the spark back to your bedroom.

It's time for you to become a fantastic partner who is not only well versed in the ancient and modern versions of the Kama Sutra techniques but a near expert on how to pleasure and treasure your partner!

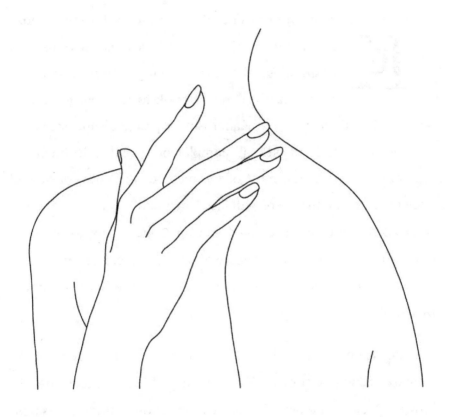

Chapter 1

What is the Kamasutra

Kama Sutra is one of the most well-known books about the history of desire, lovemaking, positioning, and other sexual practices. The Kama Sutra wasn't merely a book to read but more of a way of life. Following the Kama Sutras practices and steps led one down a path of sexual completeness and fulfillment in relationships. Although most of the methods are now considered ancient, a lot of them are still used in today's society. Though some of the practices are dated and no longer apply to modern-day, American, and European relationships, there are plenty of different parts of the world that still use the Kama Sutra and abide by every law religiously.

The Kama Sutra, though primarily a sexual-based book, actually spends most of the book talking of the origins of desire, how to woos each other, how to treat one another in relationships, etc. There is only a small section of the book allotted to sexual positioning and sexual intercourse, which most people don't realize. A lot of the time, people assume the Kama Sutra to be a book that is crude and focused solely on sex and different positions to help men and women ejaculate quicker, but this couldn't be further from the truth.

The Kama Sutra defines sexual intercourse as a divine union between man and woman. According to its author, the Hindu holy man Vatsya yana, sex in itself is not wrong. *Bad sex*, on the other hand, is not only shameful but sinful as well. Acquiring skills between the sheets is your right. It is also your duty. You owe it to yourself and to your significant other to be the best lover that you can be.

The wisdom of the Kama Sutra was once reserved only for royalty. The teachings within were exclusively taught to the ruling classes to help them achieve the perfect balance between their social and spiritual duties and living a pleasurable existence. Now, this ancient knowledge is being offered to you. This book will unveil the list of the best sex positions straight from the Kama Sutra.

According to the Kama Sutra, some sex positionsmust be performed with care as they may cause one to suffer from temporary and permanent physical injuries. Before exploring more advanced sex positions from the Kama Sutra, you must first condition your body through rigorous exercises for stamina, endurance, and flexibility. The positions included in this book are specifically designed for beginners. Simply put, you don't need to be an acrobat to make these love moves. Included are step-by-step

13

guides on how to perform each position correctly, safely, and pleasurably.

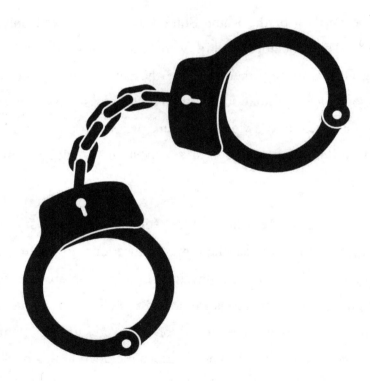

History of the Kama Sutra

The exact date that the Kama Sutra was written is not known. Still, estimates place it anywhere between 400 BCE and 300 CE. What we do know, however, is that it was officially compiled and turned into the book that we knew today in the 2nd century, otherwise known as 2 CE. This does not mean though that the book has not undergone revisions since then, and some scholars believe that the version we have is closely linked to the 3rd century, as some of the references throughout would not have applied to the 2nd century. With the text being so old, exact dating is virtually impossible. Nevertheless, there is a lot of information we do know about it.

We do know that the text originates from India, although the exact location is unknown. Historians have been able to narrow down the areato somewhere within the north or northwest region, but beyond that, it is a guess as to where the author was from. As for the author himself, we do know it was written by a man named Vatsyayana Mallanaga, as his name is engraved into the beginning of the text. Who this man was is unclear, but we do have information as to why he wrote the Kama Sutra?

Since it's a compilation in the 2nd-3rd century, the Kama Sutra has undergone numerous translations, and there are versions in almost every language. It was originally written in Sanskrit, an ancient Indian language, and this is the language that many Hindu scriptures were written in. While some translations are entirely accurate, it is important to note that some translators did place their own bias into their work, and that can be seen in the discrepancies that were later found. One of the critical examples of this was in the 19th century when the Kama Sutra was translated into English. The translator at that time wanted to ensure that the role of women in the sexual realm was not as prominent, as that was not the culture of the times. To maintain that societal understanding of sex and women, the Kama Sutra was altered so that women were significantly downplayed throughout. This has since been corrected, but it is essential to be aware of this if you ever decide to pick up a copy for yourself as you want to be sure you are getting a purer translation.

The foundations of the Kama Sutra are rooted within the Vedic Era of literature, which is based on the word Vedas. Vedas were historical texts written in India around this time that dealt with lifestyle and how one should conduct themselves daily. All works of this period were verbally passed down, and traditions were later adapted into many of the Hindu beliefs that are now practiced today. In the Vedic Era, there were distinct classes and castes within society, and a lot of that is reflected within the

Kama Sutra. Many references are made to those who are in differing classes, and how relationships between individuals of different castes cannot work out. While this type of information is not meaningful in today's culture, it does cross over when we look at socio-economic statuses and how the rich and poor interact even today.

These foundations are incredibly important because they shape the mind frame of the author of the Kama Sutra. Without grasping the history, you cannot possibly understandwhat is being discussed, as many of the terms and concepts no longer exist or are practiced currently.

It is with this in mind that we can start to see that the Kama Sutra is a religious text by some accounts. We may not associate sex and religion as being intertwined. Still, Vatsyayana saw sex as being a religious experience as well as a requirement to live a proper life. The basis of the entire viewpoint stems from certain religious beliefs, and the foundation for the whole of the book comes from his personal, religious beliefs. It is a celebration of human sexuality and the most sensual of pleasures, which are gifts from the gods and ultimately a necessity in life.

Philosophy of the Kama Sutra

As we said, we do know a bit about why Vatsyayana wrote the Kama Sutra. Looking at ancient Hindu texts, we know that the four virtues were commonly discussed and written at length about. Many of the texts focused on the two important virtues of Dharma (morality), and Athra (prosperity), while few delved into the importance of Kama (pleasure). Vatsyayana meditated upon this reality and concluded that the Kama was as important as the other virtues. So it was only proper to have a guide written solely about how to obtain the Kama.

The four virtues can be looked at more like goals that each person much work towards within their lifetime to lead a complete and fulfilled life. Within the Kama Sutra, there are many references to the other virtues as they are all tied together and must be achieved to succeed. One cannot merely focus on the physical pleasures and ignore the need for morality or prosperity so that you may notice throughout that sex and morality are often combined, as well as sex and finding a partner that brings about monetary prosperity.

To understand the philosophy behind the Kama Sutra, you must understand what it was intended to be. The sex acts that are

18

described throughout are little more than theatrics, with an emphasis on outrageous and yoga-inspired poses. The goal was unlikely to be used as a literal manual, but instead to be used as a way to understand both society and the individual. A vast majority of the book is taken up by discussing how men and women interact within society, both as a whole and simply with each other. It can be seen as almost a screenplay, taking us on a journey of love within ancient Indian times. There is talk of love, intimacy, and mundane tasks such as bathing and grooming. The Kama Sutra is a manual on all aspects of pleasure, both in the sexual sense and in the day to day realm.

The Kama is so often seen as something less important than other aspects of human pursuit. We are told to work hard, earn money, find a spouse, have children, and live a moral and righteous life. But rarely are advised on how to let loose and enjoy ourselves, or how important of a role sex plays in the human experience. The Kama Sutra is the bridge over that gap, intended to lift the importance of pleasure and sex, and place it in as high of regard as all the other aspects we are expected to work towards.

Some have questioned whether or not the Kama Sutra is a female positive as it may appear, but if you approach it from the idea of the times, then it can be seen as more of a feminist work of art than the surface would suggest.

There is obvious sexual freedom that is discussed within, one in which even our current societal viewpoint doesn't always acknowledge. Try bringing up the topic of female masturbation and see the sudden puritanical view that many people rush to. Movies are quick to showcase men sexually, but female sexuality is much more often subdued or entirely removed from the narrative. To have a book that explores the different facets of a woman's sexuality is unique, both historically as well as in the current climate. Given that the Kama Sutra talks almost nothing of procreation, it truly highlights the idea that this is a guide for pleasure and nothing more. So, by its very nature, it is also a book dedicated to a woman's desire, both by herself and that which is given to her by her partner. Beyond just sex, the Kama Sutra also discusses how to treat a woman properly so that she is nurtured and cared for in all aspects of life. It discusses showering her with affection and gifts and giving her absolute power when it comes to the home's finances.

From a philosophical standpoint, the Kama Sutra opens our minds to the needs of both men and women, and it does a good job of including women in the discussion, especially for the times. Not only does it take a more liberal and open-minded approach to women, but that same approach is extended to homosexuality and bisexuality as well. There are many references and discussions about men sleeping with men, and women pleasuring other women, as well as advice on having threesomes and even orgies.

Whatever the sexual desire is of the individual is both encouraged and celebrated, and there is no judgment cast upon those who may differ from what is considered the norm.

The Kama Sutra makes us think by challenging our conceptions and internalized beliefs when it comes to sex. Whether it is something we partake in or not, it opens our eyes to the different forms of relationships that can exist both romantically and sexually and offers up advice on how to succeed in achieving absolute pleasure. It removes the idea that sex should be for procreating and instead emphasizes the pleasure that can be found within a sexual encounter. On a deeper level, it challenges the notion that physical pleasure should take a backseat to otherworldly pursuits, and that pleasure is just as important in life as everything else. For a life without desire, it isn't truly a life worth living at all.

What Does it Teach Us?

The Kama Sutra teaches us many things, from how to take care of ourselves, to how to take care of our partner. Everything begins with you, and how you groom yourself and carry yourself in this world. It is an extremely practical guide that mixes real-world advice with philosophical ideas and concepts. It is meant to make us sit back and think about why we do what we do and how we can live a better life overall. But all of that begins with the person.

Even if we only look at the sexual aspect of the Kama Sutra, we can see exactly what the author is attempting to teach us about physical pleasure. None of us would exist without sex, so why do we diminish its role in our lives? The joyof the senses is necessary for life, so why not enjoy that and learn how to act upon those desires in both a free and moral way.

Beyond the sexual nature of the Kama Sutra, it also is a guide that teaches us how to live a good life in general. It goes in-depth on topics such as the arts, music, and literature, as well as how to be a good husband or wife. It discusses financial matters, matters of the home, and even how to properly select a spouse that is balanced with you. It goes into great detail about how you should bathe and groom yourself, where you can meet people, and how to enjoy your day and please your spouse.

From a philosophical viewpoint, it teaches us that both men and women should engage in sensual pleasures, and that sex is not just for men to get off with. Unlike many historical texts that downplay a woman's sexual desires, the Kama Sutra takes an in-depth look at what a woman's sexual nature is and how to satisfy it both before sex as well as during accurately. That isn't to say, however, that the Kama Sutra is an extremely liberal book or that it holds men and women in the same regard. It is written during a time of caste systems and where women's role in a marriage was not as high as that of the man. Men were still considered the head of the household, and much of what is described revolves around a man pursuing a woman. But, compared with other forms of literature, it does take a more liberal view of women's sexuality, as well as homosexual relationships, and the idea of having sex solely for pleasure and outside of marriage.

How to Use the Kama Sutra?

The Kama Sutra can be used in two ways, both as a practical guide as well as a philosophical work of art. Some may approach the Kama Sutra only as a guide to sex positions, and this is perfectly acceptable as a large chunk of text is dedicated to this pursuit. However, to use the Kama Sutra fully, you must look at it as a whole and take into account both the historical significance as well as the idea that it may not be as practical as one may initially think.

Many of the sex acts described within the Kama Sutra are outside an average person's ability and require a high degree of flexibility to perform. There are even positions within the book that are physically impossible unless the man has a very uniquely shaped lingam (penis). Later in this book, we will look at some of the positions that are possible, however, and break down how exactly you can do them and incorporate them into your personal sex life. In many ways, there are several similarities between the sex acts within this book and the practice of yoga. Through breathing as one with your partner, folding into different positions, and experiencing everything in unity, you can achieve a higher sense of awareness and satisfaction. So, even if you are unable to achieve the positions as described, think of it more like a workout for the mind and body and attempt a sexier form of yoga.

Since the positions are not always practical, you should use the Kama Sutra more as a general guide for how to deepen your pleasure. This book has taken many of the important concepts and ideas and broken them down into practical tips and advice so that you can elevate your sex life and truly engage in a more pleasurable and sensual experience. Beyond just the sexual side of it all, the Kama Sutra should also be used as a guide on how to treat your partner both inside and outside of the bedroom. It can assist you in being more romantic and intimate, as well as teach you how to make sure your partner is entirely satisfied within the relationship.

With a breakdown of different personalities and temperaments, the Kama Sutra also discusses how you can go about finding the right partner for you based on ancient concepts and ideas. While some of the information may seem absurd in the context of today's world, not everything should be taken as a literal word. Instead, it is vital that you read the Kama Sutra as a concept more than a script and that between the lines, you see that even the most ancient of dating tips are still applicable today.

Chapter 2

Love with Kamasutra

The idea that the Kama Sutra is all about contorted sexual positions and the physicality of sensual pleasures is extremely erroneous. The Kama Sutra is so much more than that, and anyone who has ever tried, or at least read up on the ways of the best-known Sutra, will tell you it's an education in itself.

The creation of the Kama Sutra by its authors was to make partners understand and use the sexual energy between them into something meaningful, spiritual, and healthy. It is unfortunate that many of the present-day authors and commentators only focus on the physical aspect of the Kama Sutra.

It has been widely misunderstood and misrepresented. Kama Sutra goes far deeper than just explosive orgasms and insatiable sexual appetites.

In its most basic principle, the Kama Sutra was served to make couples happy and in effect, make the relationship stronger. The Kama Sutra was designed to make both men and women aware of the pleasures of the flesh as well as pleasure on an intellectual level. It's not just a sex tip book.

The Kama Sutra originally included topics like About the Wives of Other Men, Society, and Social Concepts, About the Acquisition of a Wife, about a Wife, On Sexual Union, About Courtesans, and On the Means of Attracting Others to Yourself and About Courtesans.

The book is explicit on details on how to win the mind and body of a woman and what a woman should do to win the man. It explores the states of a woman's thinking (insert pun), the role that a go-between plays in a relationship as well as why would a woman turn down a man's advances.

Kama Sutra also discusses the points of whether you choose a childhood friend to have a relationship with over colleagues.

Some illustrations and charts would emphasize the characteristics and the different physical types of bodies and how this affects the compatibility of the couple.

The Kama Sutra also illustrates the many varieties of embraces, kissing, oral sex, and sexual intercourse. And not so surprisingly, a list of instructions about extramarital affairs and how to conduct relationships with the 'wives of other men.'

There are also pages devoted to scratching and biting, and on how these can excite lovemaking. The book also talks about dealings with courtesans and their styles of seduction and how you can spot their extortion methods.

What the Kama Sutra Says About Love

The Kama Sutra discusses love in-depth and focuses heavily on marriages as the best type of union. With that said, however, it does acknowledge that not all sexual relations happen within the confines of marriage, and it does discuss the varying types of relationships that can occur. While you should never be something you are not just to please someone else, the idea of working on your personality and qualities to enhance them and make yourself more attractiveis certainly not a negative. We should all work towards building up who we are, being confident in ourselves, and feeling free enough to express our innermost desires.

Physical Attraction and Love

Although love requires much more than a simple physical attraction, the way a person looks is frequently the first thing that draws us to them. When you are looking to meet someone, and you know nothing about them as a person, you are going solely off of how they look to you. If someone is physically unattractive in your eyes, there is very little chance that you will want to pursue something intimate with them, and thus the road to love is cut short.

Love by Continual Habit

Love by continual habit is described in the Kama Sutra as the love that comes from repetition and practice of an act. In a non-romantic way, this is the love that may develop for a specific hobby as you continue to practice it and get better at it. The more you engage yourself and learn, the more you develop a love and passion. Romantically, this is the love that develops over a long time with an individual, either within or outside of a romantic relationship. For example, some people may begin as friends long before they become lovers. Over time, as they do activities together, engage in long, in-depth talks, and grow as people, they eventually fall in love. This is the continual habit of being around someone and continuing to learn about them and grow together as a couple. This is a solid form of love, as there is an excellent foundation to it, and it is built not on lust but entirely on love.

Love by Imagination

Love by imagination is in complete contrast to love by continual habit, as it is far from physical and exists purely within the mind. This is the type of love that has no bearing in the real world and instead is created within a fantasy of your choosing. An innate kindof love, it is one that already exists within you and requires no effort or forming of habits to induce. It is a type of love that exists before your partner and will continue to exist despite your partner as they do not create it. It can, however, be influenced and informed by your partner, but for the most part, it is merely an innate feeling that you have.

Love from Belief

Love from belief is a love that is understood by both parties and is something felt deep within ourselves. It is the type of love in which we have no questions, no doubts, and no fears. When we genuinely believe in love, when we believe in our feelings, we know that it is accurate and real. This is one of the most potent forms of love, and it is the one in which meaningful relationships are built upon. Love from belief stems from excellent communication, high levels of trust, and mutual understanding that you both have developed with time and care. It stems from years of work, as well as effort and actions purposely used to cr

eate it.

Love Created from the Perception of External Objects

Within the Kama Sutra, this is considered the highest form of love, and all other types of love are there only to lead to and enhance this. This is the love you feel for what is in front of you, and it is a tangible form of love based upon what you can see and feel. All of the types we discussed above are based on this, as each is used as a way to feel, show, and create a love for that which is external to yourself. How you see something and experience, it is going to develop and shape your love for it, and without an external source, there honestly is nothing to love.

Benefits of Kama Sutra and Sex Kama Sutra will bring you closer together.

This is all about experimentation here, which Is a wild and beautiful thing. It states that if both partners take a sense of humor about it and laugh it off together when a position goes wrong or

needs practice, then you get closer.

Kama Sutra values empowering women

Despite all that our modern-day society keeps preaching about women and sexuality, Kama Sutra has a different view on this subject matter. Kama Sutra suggests that a woman needs to study the variousforms of sex before she gets married. When a woman understands the different forms of sex, she would be a better mate and would be more desirable by her man. So, the Kama Sutra encouraging women and empowering them is one of the most significant benefits you stand to gain from the book.

Kama Sutra

makes a clear classification of a man's penis

Also, the Kama Sutra made mention of the size of a man's penis and that it matters when choosing a mate. There are three types of man penis by Kama Sutra – the bull, horse, and hare. Kama Sutra also made mention of different sizes of woman's vagina, and that a perfect match of the vagina size and penis sizes would result in an excellent sexual experience.

Kama Sutra also emphasizes on living a healthy life and well-balanced one

Kama Sutra is also a book that talks about tips on how to live a healthy life. The Kama Sutra encourages that a man and a woman should embrace cleanliness, which would, in turn, boost their health. A man, for instance, should shave his beard regularly, and take his bath and eat healthily, and the same applies to a woman too. She should bread her hair and shave as well. Couples could also try mutual grooming.

Kama Sutra talks about enticing and approaching women

The Kama Sutra also talks about exciting tips a man can use to entice and approaching a woman. This tip helps men to know how to touch and caress a woman in other to express their desire when they want to have sex. When a man knows these various tips and how to use them, he will find it easier to get his message over to the woman. The suggestions of how to entice and approach a woman further move on to touching and embracing.

Kama Sutra talks about eight different types of embrace

There are different types of embrace from the Kama Sutra. It further tells us that there are up to eight different types of embrace thatcan be used for different purposes. Because of Kama Sutra's teaching, we now know how to apply the various types of embrace. And applying the right type of embrace at the right moment would set the right mood in motion. So, rather than keeping all your emotions inside, you can now use the various teaching from Kama Sutra about embrace to seduce and lure your lover into that perfect love zone.

Kama Sutra teaches about kissing

There are different forms of kissing too. Kama Sutra also teaches that a woman should feel too shy about a kiss. We all know that a man, in most cases, is the ones that initiate the kiss, but a woman should not feel shy to be the one to start the kiss first. There are also different types of kiss that partners can use to connect at particular points in your relationship deeply. Like a kindof kissing, couples can engage in when walking on a lonely street. There are also different types of kiss that lovers can engage in when they want to make love.

Kama Sutra is divided into a set of 64 acts

Contrary to the belief that the Kama Sutra doesn't have a list of sex positions howbeit lovemaking that includes penetration is divided into 64 acts. This act explains the different ways couples can have sex to enjoy the maximum pleasure from sex. To have the best sex, you have to combine it with stimulating desire and engaging in an embrace, caressing, kissing, biting, slapping, moans, oral sex, and everything in-between.

Kama Sutra recommends that your scratch your partner

There are different types of scratch you can have with your partner. With this knowledge Kama Sutra provides us, we can add a twist to lovemaking without loved ones. Moreover, leaving scratch marks on your lover's body can help keep the fire burning for each other even when your lover is not close to you.

Kama Sutra recommends that your woman lover should reach orgasm first

When making love with our loved once, Kama Sutra suggests that the woman should be the first to have an orgasm. This point is valid because of the extreme exhaustion a man feels after having an orgasm, whereby he wouldn't be able to proceed with sex at least not immediately. So, in other to have great sex, the woman should be the first to have an orgasm before the man allows himself to have an orgasm.

Kama Sutra also talks about a woman's sex as being more than just sex penetrations

In Kama Sutra, there is more to sex than penetration for a woman. To a woman, the whole act is sensual, but a man reaches orgasm at the end of the intercourse. Most men think that making a woman have an orgasm is their ultimate act, but a woman needs both sexual and physiological pleasure to be able to satisfy her urge. Thanks to Kama Sutra, many men who were getting this concept wrong have been able to make adjustments.

The Kama Sutra teaches you the art of fellatio and cunnilingus

Most people have a way of approaching oral sex, which is what is described above in the subtitle, in the same old way. This is a common thing, and a lot of times, it's taken as a job with skills that are not that good because face it, most of us have no one to teach us, and the only role model they have is porn, which is fantasy at best.

Kama Sutra makes you so much more confident

Being a great lover and partner and seeing the look on your partner's face will give you a huge confidence boost. When you're more confident doing one of the most nerve-wracking things and the thing that makes you the most vulnerable because you are naked, then you can do anything.

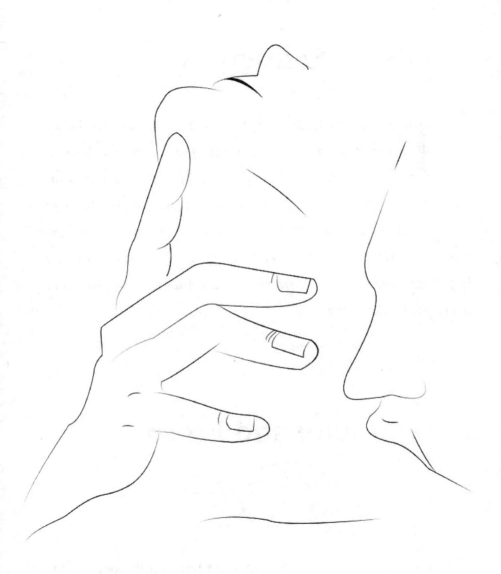

Chapter 3

Seduction

The actions leading up to the sex part is every bit as important as the sex itself. Guys, there's nothing pleasurable about simply shoving your tool in your partner and hoping she gets off when you get off. While guys have it relatively easy when it comes to sexual arousal and orgasms, girls take a little longer to heat up. This is why it's important to set the mood just right and get a girl good, wet, and ready before doing the deed.

Clean and Fresh

If a guy wants a girl to go down on him – a thorough bath, scrubbing all the parts that need to be cleansed, should be performed before anything else. It's only polite, and the clean smell makes women more eager to hit all those erogenous spots.

Ladies, this goes both ways. If you want a guy to pay attention to the body hotspots and linger on the foreplay, it matters very much to be clean and fresh. This is especially true if you're hoping for some oral sex. A lot of males also prefer their women to be clean-cut down under since it makes everything more comfortableand more pleasurable to the tongue. More on that will be discussed later.

Dirty Talk

It is usually the males who love dirty talk, but women also find it arousing. The concept of dirty talk is pretty blurry, but for the most part, this involves being explicit about what you want or what you feel. For example, a girl might be straightforward in telling a guy that she wants his cock in her mouth or his mouth, suckling her breasts. It may also involve complimenting a guy about his length or girth as he penetrates. The words 'cock', 'cunt', and 'pussy' are relatively common in dirty talk and often used in placeof the terms penis and vagina.

Bedroom Games

If you've heard of 50 Shades of Grey, you'll have a pretty good idea about bedrom games and how you can make the sex more exciting. Roleplay is a relatively common way of keeping things exciting and can offer some of the most mind-blowing sexual encounters between you and your partner. The use of toys would also be helpful. In a later chapter, you'll find out more about sex toys and how to best utilize them to keep each other satisfied.

Porn

This is a grey area for most couples. While guys have no problem getting a hard-on while watching porn, some women will need a longer time to get aroused. However, watching porn does help set the stage when it comes to sex, letting your partner get the message as soon as the scene starts to play.

When it comes right down to it, there are lots of things couples can do to set the mood for sex. From the vanilla to the alarming, what's important about preludes to sex is that both partners find it arousing and are 100% consensual about the whole thing.

A Sight to Remember

The visual experience of sex is one of the most important ones. Particularly for men as they are visual creatures who rely heavily on what they see to turn them on and get them in the mood. Because of this, you'll want to make sure that wherever you're having sex doesn't have too many visual disturbances. For example, a messy or overly bright/clashing room might make for too much to look at, causing you guys to become distracted and ruin the tone. Additionally, dirty rooms can cause clutter to get in the way of you two. It is a good idea to tidy up the area you intend to have sex in.

Smells like Roses

Well, you don't exactly have to smell like roses, though they are a delightful and romantic smell. But you do want to make sure that the sense of smell is added into the tone-setting mix. Setting this part is easy: melt soe wax in a delicious warm scent (such as vanilla or berry), wear a small amount cologne or perfume, use freshly washed sheets. You want to make sure the area, and you, smell enticing.

Touch Me

Physical touch is another incredibly significant portion of setting the tone. The type of physical touch we're talking about doesn't involve touching of the genitals, though a little "accidental" brush of the hand never hurt anyone. But what you want to do is make sure you're stimulating their boy: press your thigh into theirs when you sit on the couch, hold their knee under the table, hold hands on the way home, hug each other extra-long before you sit down, stroke the other person's hair while you tell them you love them. You want to stimulate their body to make them feel physically wanted by you, but in an innocent way. This is a wonderful way to set the intimacy, even in everyday experiences where you aren't trying to set the tone for sex.

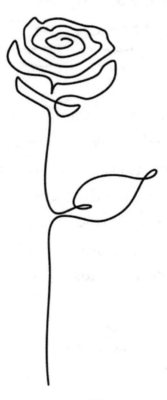

Chapter 4 Intimacy

Intimacy, in a general sense, is defined as mutual openness and vulnerability. There are different ways that intimacy can show up in a relationship, as long as it involves giving and receiving vulnerability. Different, more specific types of intimacy are present in different relationships. In this chapter, we will focus on two of these forms of intimacy-emotional intimacy and physical intimacy.

Emotional Vs. Physical Intimacy

Emotional intimacy is the ability to express oneself maturely and openly, which leads to a deep emotional connection between two people. Saying things like "I love you" or "you are critical to me" are examples of this. It is also the ability to respond maturely and openly when someone expresses themselves to you by saying things like "I'm sorry" or "I love you too." This type of intimacy is found in romantic relationships, and some friendships or familial relationships.

Physical intimacy is the type of intimacy that most people think of when they hear the term, and it is the kind that we have been addressing the most so far in this book. This is the type of intimacy that includes physical touch, including sex and all activities related to sex. However, it also involves other non-sexual types of physical contact, such as hugging and kissing.

How to Increase Intimacy

In a romantic or sexual relationship, intimacy is a given. You would not enter a romantic relationship without some degree of emotional intimacy, and a sexual relationship by definition involves physical intimacy. For a romantic relationship to be successful, both forms of intimacy must be present between the partners. Without intimacy, there is nothing that sets a romantic relationship apart from an everyday friendship. Intimacy is something that must be worked at and maintained consistently, especially emotional intimacy. In a romantic relationship, however, physical intimacy must be maintained as well as this is one way of showing the other person that you feel strongly for them. If intimacy is lacking or if it fades over time, there are some things that you can do to revive or rekindle it.

The first way to restore intimacy in a relationship or to develop it in the first place is through communication. Communication is key in a relationship of any sort, but especially in a romantic relation. Communicating is the only sure way to know where the other person stands in terms of their thoughts and feelings. Being able to be vulnerable and open with your emotions is a requirement for intimacy. It is necessary to share oneself with the other person in a relationship. This mutual sharing of yourselves is what will lead to intimacy in the first place or an increase in intimacy.

It is important to communicate about your needs for intimacy repeatedly since people will grow and change throughout a relationship. Especially in a long-term relationship, being aware of when a person's intimacy needs change is important to maintaining therightlevel of intimacy.

When working on intimacy, it is helpful to start slow by talking about things that are easier for you to open up about-like your future goals or your ideal job. This is still a way to open up without pushing yourself too far right away. It can be scary to be that vulnerable with someone. It is also helpful to note that for many people, there are things that they consciously avoid thinking about, as they may be painful to address. It will be challenging for them to voice these things to themselves, so allow them to start slowly and don't be offended if you feel like there are topics that they are uncomfortable talking about.

Many people have a fear of intimacy, and this is also worth noting. Because intimacy needs trust to develop, it can be hard for some people who have had past experiences that make it hard for them to trust people. By being aware of this, it may help you to understand why your partner has trouble opening up. It may also help you if you have a fear of intimacy as you can explain this to your partner to ask for the patience you will need as you begin to open up and be vulnerable with them.

When it comes to improving intimacy, it is a slow build and not a race to the finish line. Be patient with yourself and your partner, and try to see intimacy as a growing experience between you that will continue throughout the entire duration of your relationship.

The Art of Kissing

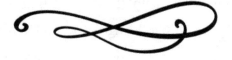

When kissing comes to mind, one might imagine that the act of locking lips should be pretty straightforward. After all, kissing has been regarded as a symbol of love, seemingly since the beginning of humanity. It's typically the first indication that a relationship is progressing to a more romantic level. When done correctly, it should send both parties into a state of passion, desire, and excitement.

Kissing is seen as something that should occur before sex, and Vatsyayana was a firm believer that actions such as kissing, embracing, and scratching are not meant to be used during sexual intercourse. Instead, these are all different forms of foreplay, and as such, should be engaged in to arouse our partner and prepare them for a sexual union.

The Power of Touch

It has been said that sexual intercourse, when done correctly, can be compared with the simplest of things like building a sandcastle. For it not to fall, it must have a strong base put in place.

In can then be built up slowly and finished with some fine sculpting and nurturing to bring out its full beauty. Once enjoyed and marveled at it can be allowed to be washed away slowly and returned to a natural position.

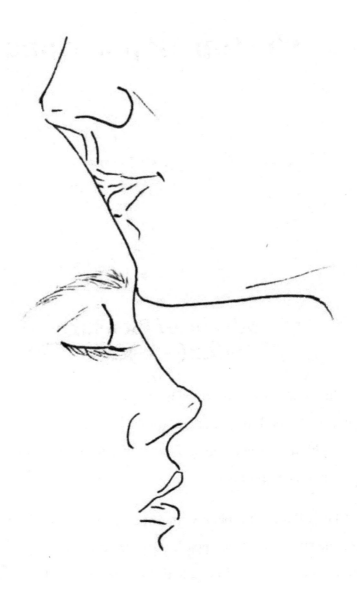

Chapter 5

The top 18 positions

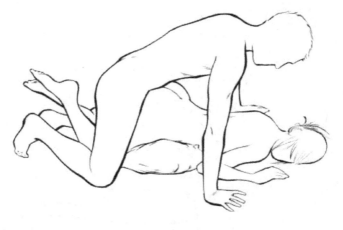

Mirror of Pleasure

This is a complete position for young lovers to practice and develop. It is both physical and romantic as the man takes his lady from behind, but she can look at him adoringly while accepting his lingam deep into her.

She is flat on her back with arms by her sides but entices him with the majesty of her pearl, so it requires him to lift her legs high and to the side. He can lean forward here and put one strong arm down by her side to keepeye contact between lovers.

She can enjoy his powerful chest while feeling his lingam push profoundly and meaningfully into her. They can even hold hands on one side while with one arm, he holds both legs as if holding open a curtain for her to join him in the same chamber. The mirror forms the perfect setting for our two lovers to look starry-eyed at each other.

Merger

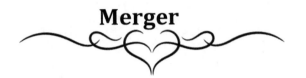

The position sees both lovers sit back on the mat on the floor, supporting themselves with their arms back and hands behind them. They can look at each other and cross their legs until the crouch can touch one another's.

The woman can use her flexibility to position her yoni over his erection. She should comfortably sit on his penis and lift her body with her hands. She can contort her torso back and forth on his shaft, and her yoni should be open to penetration but lower to the ground.

This can be very pleasurable as the walls of her vagina stroke up and down his penis. She must makemost of the rocking motion, but she is a fee to conduct how fast the action needs to be.

As you can see, they will be in a complete merger of bodies as they intertwine until orgasm.

Speed Bump

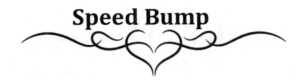

The speed bump is an excellent technique that enters from behind and can also be used for anal sex. It is a unique position for slow and sensual sex while he nibbles on your back or neck, or for faster sex where he can wildly thrust until you both orgasms. Due to the angle of penetration, it stimulates several areas within' the vagina that are typically missed from front-facing positions. It works by having the lady lay on her tummy with her legs tightly closed together, and her arms tucked in underneath her. Then, the gentleman slides on top of her and enters her from behind. Having her legs locked tight can increase the sensations, as it makes it easier to contract around his penis and create a tighter entry for him, making it more pleasurable for both lovers.

Edge of Heaven

The edge of heaven positions uses a chair, bed, or couch to create heaven's edge. This is an excellent position for the female orgasm, as it creates deep penetration, and her sensual areas are mainly supporting her. To start, the gentleman should sit on the edge of a seat with his feet on the floor. Then, the lady should straddle on top of him on his lap, with a leg on either side of him. The gentleman should then hold underneath her knees while keeping her legs up in the air, and the lady can balance herself on his lap. He can now thrust as deep and quick as he desires while stimulating her g-spot and driving her to an incredible orgasm.

Magic Bullet

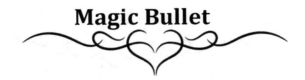

This position is another phenomenal one for deep penetration and stimulating the g-spot. It is a man-dominant position that is excellent for her pleasure and orgasm. It starts by having the lady lying on her back on the bed. She can either support her head with the bed or hang her head over the edge of the bed. Then, the gentleman can sit on his knees, spread them wide open, and scooch in close so he can penetrate her. She can put her legs straight up in the air, so the backs of her legs rest on his chest, and he can use her legs for leverage to thrust. For added pleasure and stimulation, she can rub her clitoris to help her achieve orgasm.

Jellyfish

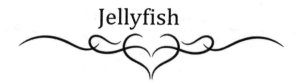

This position is very affectionate and places the lovers face to face to speak and kiss each other fondly. The man should sit upright on a mat and the floor and welcome himover onto his lap.

She can massage his penis slowly and purposefully until he gets a full erection. She can always take his erection in her mouth and suck him until he is fully hard and ready.

She then gently gets onto his lap and allows for full or half penetration. She can choose to take his penis to massage her clitoris or take penetration into her yoni and move back and forth.

She is in full facial position in front of him, and her breasts are open to his playfulness.

Possession

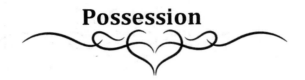

This is an exciting position because it will involve his lingam entering her from an unusual angle. The starting position is one where she accepts him when lying flat on her back. She keeps her legs well apart, but he enters her from a sitting position keeping his legs forward and under her arms.

Here he can grasp her arms firmly and pull her body down onto his erection while thrusting his lower abdomen forward, maximizing as much as possible his sitting position.

Because of the angle of her hip bone, his lingam will be forced downwards onto the lower section of her vagina walls, giving her an altogether different experience. Her pearl is wide open to some stimulation with his fingers, and she can have a double penetration type experience.

Arms of Mill

This position may come as a completely new and novel experience for many. It is another position where the actual penetration will feel very different to the norm. The woman will lie down on her back and comfortably places her legs wide apart to allow her man full access.

This he does willingly, but the Arms of Mill require him to lie face down with his head pointing away from here.

Here the lovers do not see eye to eye in true Yab-Yum fashion because when she reaches down, she will be presented with his buttocks to massage. His penetration will again be felt quite differently in her yoni and is a pleasurable experience.

The lack of movement available is more than made up for by the various parts of the body each lover can reach with their spare hand. He could reach under and finger her anus while she could likewise do the same simultaneously.

Slept

The Slept is another position best performed on the ground, and as the man lays behind his woman, he can take her leg behind him the same way as shownduring the Dragonfly. This time, to make penetration, a natural act is for him to pull his leg over her prostate leg, meaning he controls her pelvic region and can maximize his entrance into her.

With her free leg held out of the way, he can freely thrust his pelvis, making his lingam a battering ram of love.

She can enjoy the sensation of deep penetration and the feeling of being taken from behind at the same time. He also gets to massage her back and bite her neck of kiss her breast giving her many simultaneous pleasures.

Pushcart

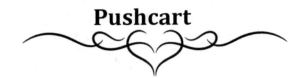

This is a relatively straight forward position as long as the lady can maintain her upper body weight if her legs are lifted off the floor. Her man can do this while she lays on the floor or bed, and as the name would suggest, he picks up her quivering thighs and can spread them wide apart, leaving her anticipating pearl at his complete disposal.

The thought of this openness and vulnerability is a complete turn-on for many women, and he is obliged to make his penetration as lasting and memorable as the chance he has been given.

If she has a supple back, she can throw her head back in wild celebration of the treatment she is receiving, and the original shopping cart awkwardness of their opening move will soon be forgotten.

Screw

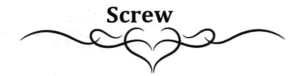

This is not just an easy acronym for sexual intercourse but involves a very flexible screwing position by the lady. She is required to twist her abdomen entirely around, so her shoulders stay on the edge of her bed, but her pearl is exposed in all its glory, waiting for his eager services.

From here, he can quickly provide his thrust into her anus, giving this positon a feeling of wildness and forcefulness if she can manage to turn and open up.

Sultry Saddle

This position is a wonderful one for anyone who is looking for something new to spice up the bedroom life. It works by having the gentleman lie down on his back, with his knees bent and his legs apart. The lady can then nuzzle in between his legs and achieve penetration. Using one hand on his chest and another on his leg, you can rock yourselves out of this world. The benefit of the woman being on top is that she can control the depth and where she's being stimulated, while the man can lay back and enjoy the ride.

The Squat

This woman-on-top position is perfect for the lady to pick the speed, rhythm, and angle. The man can still use his hands and thrusting action, however, to gain a little control for himself as well. The gentleman lies on his back on the bed with his knees up and separated. Then, the lady squats on top of him and rides him. You can hold each other's hands for ample thrusting leverage, or she can put her hands on his chest to gain control while he holds her hips to keep them in rhythm with each other. It is an excellent way to achieve a deep penetration that caresses the g-spot.

Face to Face

This position is an incredibly romantic position that provides an excellent angle for penetration while enabling the two lovers to make out still. It is a slower position that stimulates a more relaxing, love-making situation. It works by having the gentleman sit with his legs comfortably out in front of him, knees slightly bent and separated. Then, the lady can slide in on his lap, wrap her legs around him, and be penetrated. The angle works wonderfully for g-spot stimulation, and you can go as fast or as slow as you want to while enjoying the romantic moment with each other.

Freaky Lovers

This position is excellent for the pro-lovers who are into downright freaky sex moves. It mixes experimental, exciting moves with your desire to stand entirely outside of the box when it comes to sex. You can use these moves to make for a hot bedroom encounter, blowing each other's mind one thrust at a time. Use these moves to enhance your experience, stimulate ultimate pleasure, and create incredibly intimate and romantic intercourse as you explore each other in ways you never have before.

Lotus Like Position

In the Lotus Like Position, the woman will cross her lower calves across one another to create a position similar to what is seen during a lotus style sit in yoga. While on her back, she should bring her legs up into the air, either entirely or only partially, and then place one calf over top of the other. For a more traditional pose, her legs should be partially lifted, which can be achieved by having her start with her legs bent but feet planted on the ground. From here, all she needs to do it lift her feet off the ground and then raise her lower legs until she can comfortably cross them. The man will find it most comfortableto approach this position from a kneeling position, and he should also noticethat her feet naturally fall against his chest. By keeping the woman's feet on his chest, he can not only support her, but he can use his body weight to push her legs backward, making it easier for him to reach her vagina.

For women that are very flexible, or who would like to practice this in a very traditional way, you should cross the legs like you are in a seated position. To get an idea of what this means, start this position by being seated on your buttocks, and then cross your legs over each other as if you were preparing to meditate. Each foot should rest on the opposite thigh, while the calves will firmly press against one another. Once you have this wholly understood, simply lay back without changing your legs at all. When your man comes to enter you, he will press your crossed legs back against you, and your feet will touch between your breasts and your stomach. As sex progresses, the man can spread the woman's legs apart when he feels necessary, switching up the angle and position freely.

Turning Position

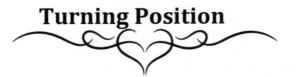

The Turning Position switches things up significantly, and it is now the man who will need to perform quite the acrobatic feat to get into this position properly. For this, the couple should start in a regular missionary style position, with the woman on her back and the man on top of her. Women will need to ensure that their legs are not bent, as the man is going to need a smooth surface to work on. Once sex is well underway, the man is going to lift himself, remain inside the woman, and then spin himself around so that he is now facing towards her feet. At no point can the man leave the woman's vagina, as he must remain inside at all times. Sound complicated? It is.

How you make, this work is going to be very much up to you, as it will significantly depend on the man's penis. His length will play a significantrole in whether or not this is even possible, as well as the direction that his erection naturally leans. If the man has an erection that is very rigid and points up towards the belly button, The Turning Position is not likely to be possible. Instead, the man needs a more flexible erection that can alter its angle as he turns. If you are not able to turn yourself around during sex without leaving the vagina, don't worry. You can always modify this pose by turning and re-entering if possible.

Supported Congress

The Supported Congress is the first of the positions we have come to that gets both partners up and off of the ground. Here is a classic standing pose that is fairly simple and is modified depending on your personal preference. To perform The Supported Congress, have both partners stand face one another. From here, you only need to find something to support you; the Kama Sutra suggests using each other's bodies, a wall, or a pillar. How you engage in sex after this point is up to you. Some options include standing with both feet on the ground and then angling the pelvis so that the man can insert himself into the woman. Another option is to have the woman raise one of her legs so that entry can be even easier.

One important thing to know with most standing positions is that height differences can make or break what you can do. In many cases, the man is going to be taller than the woman, which means their pelvic regions generally will not line up perfectly. To combat this issue, utilize things around the house to bring the woman up to a taller stance. You can try wearing high heels or standing on the lower part of your staircase if you have one. You can also stand on cushions, a small stepping stool, or anything else that is stable and gives you enough of a boost to have sex more enjoyable.

Chapter 6

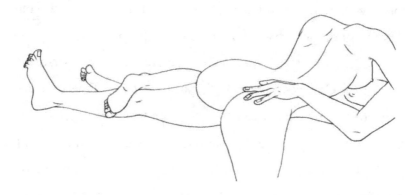

The top 10 relaxing positions

Churning

The man grabs his penis at its base. He penetrates the woman and circles the inside walls of her vagina. This isn't about deep penetration. It's about exploring the sensitivity of the woman's vaginal walls, which varies from woman to woman. The longer the penis, the better this technique will work.

Rubbing

Generally speaking, when a man is penetrating a woman, he should aim for the front wall of the vagina. That typically where a woman's g-spot will be found. But if a man were to occasionally go for the back wall with short and sharp thrusts instead of the deep plunging, he can create a very different but enjoyable experience for the woman.

One-sided Scissor

If your weight is pretty optimal, but your female partner is a bit more on the femininecurvacious side, then have her lay on her back so you can view her ample breasts before you...yum! Then, make sure her bottom in the right beyond the edge of the bed or any platform, then you are in an optimal position.

The bed or platform should reach exactly or near enough to your hip level as a man. This gives you better penetration leverage. Take one of her ankles, whichever side is more comfortable for both of you, and raise the leg so that her ankle is on your shoulder.

Penetrate her then. She may want to hold on to the sheets or blanket or the edge of the table or platform. This gives you leverage.

Two-sided Scissor

Repeat all steps on position two, but the only difference being that you grab both her ankles and place them on both your shoulders before penetration. This is slightly more comfortable, and if the gentleman is overweight, all three of these exercises work best. We will go more into weight and those factors later in the nest chapter.

Kneeling Scissor

You may also accomplish the same amount of joy in the first two scissors positions by having the male kneel in front of his voluptuous partner and penetrate her on the ground. Now, just a note about ground level, it's not going to be quite as a level between his hips to hers.

However, what needs to happen in this case is she must be as flexible as possible because he has to lean in towards her chest, and her legs on his shoulders are going to go back some. Now, you can modify this position if she isn't that flexible. Instead of her legs being on either shoulder, you can have them spread out into a V shape, and her ankles can be right by the sides of your shoulders or broader.

Another modification to make up for any lack of flexibility is going to be if the female bends her knees. This will allow her to bring her knees as far up toward her shoulders or chest as possible.

Galloping Horse

The galloping horse is an exciting, fast-paced position that allows for incredibly deep penetration. The lady has little to no control in this position, which can add to her pleasure. It requires a chair, as other seat choices will not enable the position to work correctly. To start, have the gentleman sitting down with his legs straightened and feet on the floor. Then, the lady should sit on his lap, facing him, with a leg on either side. He can then enter her while she picks her feet up off of the floor and puts them straight out behind him. He can hold her upper arms or shoulders to stop her from falling back, while also giving him leverage to thrust underneath her while she bounces on top of him. It is guaranteed to provide the ultimate deep penetration experience that will send both of you over the edge in no time.

The Good Spread

This position is best if the lady is flexible, as it requires her to have her legs stretched out straight to either side. It allows for deep penetration, and for the woman to control the speed and rhythm, as well as where he is stimulating her. The man will have free hands, so he can rub her thighs or massage her breasts while she rides him. To start, the gentleman should be lying on his back with his legs; however, he feels they are most comfortable. Then, the lady should mount him, facing him, but sitting upright. Each leg should be stretched out on either side of him, and she can lean forward slightly and use his chest to help her bounce up and down on him. Take care not to bounce out of control, as that could hurt him. Then, he can admire her while she pleasures herself on him.

The Melody Maker

This position takes control away from the female entirely and gives it to the male. It is perfect for hitting the g-spot and provides the gentleman with the ability to use his spare hand to stimulate her clitoris at the same time, ensuring she will achieve a mind-blowing orgasm. Bonus points if they both orgasm at the same time! To start, have the female lay back over a piece of furniture, with her feet firmly on the floor. Then, he can come in between her legs and penetrate her. Depending on the height of the furniture, he may or may not have to get down on his knees to be at the same height as her. He can hold her hands, stimulate her clitoris, massage her breasts, or do anything they desire.

Hit The Spot

This position is an excellent behind-entry position that allows for deep penetration and ample stimulation. It might look a bit acrobatic, but it is fantastic for both lovers' pleasure. It is a man-on-top position that almost eliminates any control from the female. To start, the lady should be on her tummy on a flat surface. Then, the gentleman should come behind her on his knees and slide his knees under her belly. He can enter her similar to doggy-style while she then wraps one of her legs around him so he can get deeper. He can put his arms next to her and use them to keep her in place.

Dashing Rider

This is a phenomenal woman-on-top position that can be altered to suit any rider. To start, you want to have the gentleman lying comfortably on his back. Then, the lady can sit on top of him, sideways. She can choose how he penetrates her, and she can ride him at her own chosen speed and rhythm. It helps her control where she is being stimulated and how. It is a comfortable position that has minimum stimulation over the clitoris and g-spot, but due to the angle makes it feel like she is getting filled full.

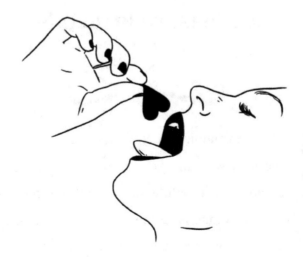

Chapter 7

The top 12 dominant positions of women

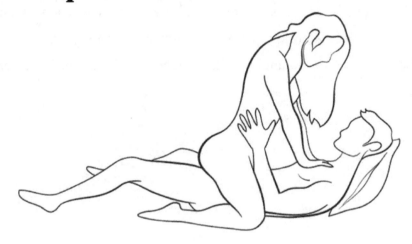

The Pleasure Principle

Before explaining techniques on how a man can please a woman, the matter of how he learns must be addressed. While some men may have a selfish approach to sex, if a woman is learning about the Kama Sutra, it's a reasonable assumption that she is with a partner who cares about her pleasure. That only leaves the question of whether or not her partner knows **how** to give her pleasure.

While learning techniques is always helpful, it is the woman's responsibility to communicate her desires and ways she enjoys being stimulated. For obvious reasons, it's to her benefit that she do so. Still, many women feel awkward or fear their partner will think them "slutty" or "cheap."This is why it's so important to use the full scope of the Kama Sutra to create a deep connection. Any feelings of awkwardness or fear judgment must be addressed.

It's not fair for a partner to be limited in how much pleasure they can get from lovemaking because they're afraid to give a voice to their desires and fantasies. It's equally unfair to leave one's lover fumbling in the dark (sometimes literally!) to find what works and doesn't work for their partner.

Great sex requires the person to feel sexy. And while being pleasured and desired can make a person feel sexy, they also need to feel they are rightand pleasing their partner.

Some men don't take criticism well. But virtually all men want to be skilled lovers. So to educate them, it might come down to how the lesson is presented more than the lesson itself.

Instead of "It doesn't feel good when you do that," try, "I've been wondering what it would feel like if you did it this way."

Instead of "You go too fast," try, "I think if we go slower, you might be able to give me an even bigger orgasm."

The suggestions don't have to be verbal. Grabbing your partner's hand and placing it where you want it, along with a heartfelt moan can be a blameless, shameless step in the right direction.

The Coital Alignment Technique

The woman lies on her back. The man lies above, as one would in the missionary position. The man positions himself higher up so that his penis enters her and points downward instead of upward—the dorsal side of the penis presses on the clitoris. Instead of thrusting upward, the man pushed downward. The woman might wrap her legs around him, but the driving movement of the lovemaking comes from the pelvises. The woman controls the upward strokes, and the man leads the downward stroke.

The Triads of Desire

Pleasuring your love with oral sex is one thing. Doing so while playing with a nipple might be even better. Are you pleasuring your partner with oral sex while playing with a nipple and slowly massaging the area around the rectum? That could send your partner into pleasure overload.

This technique is mainly usedfor couples that have been together for a long time because there are so many possible combinations. Ears, nipples, vagina, penis, rectum, thigh, belly button, or any part of the body where you know they enjoy or that you've yet to explore. To add to the unpredictability, the intensity can vary for each body part, and so can the temperature. Having a cup of ice chips nearby can come in handy.

The nipples can be stimulated in so many ways. A kiss, a flick of the tongue, sucking, a playful bite, or aggressive biting are just a few examples of varying intensities. And that's without using your hands! Add to this, the options of blowing on them or rubbing an ice chip on it. Whatever can be done to the nipple, can be done to pretty much any part of the body.

The "triads of desire" is meant to be playful and unpredictable. It's important to be aware of your partner's reactions and signals. Otherwise, you run the risk of having your points of desire to become more distraction than seduction.

The Genie Lamp

A woman is on all fours as a man takes her from behind. While performing what is commonly know as "doggie style," the man waits until the woman is getting close to climax. He reaches around her and places his hands just above her pubic bone. He rubs his hands in opposite directions. Because this area is incredibly sensitive for women, the stimulation can reach much higher levels.

Legs Up!

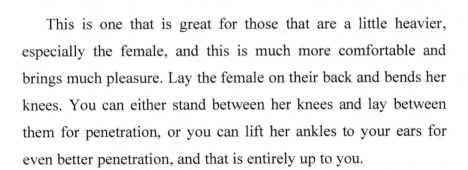

This is one that is great for those that are a little heavier, especially the female, and this is much more comfortable and brings much pleasure. Lay the female on their back and bends her knees. You can either stand between her knees and lay between them for penetration, or you can lift her ankles to your ears for even better penetration, and that is entirely up to you.

Standing Suspended

This first position is excellent for the female orgasm because of the angle that the man's penis enters her vagina and also because the man is in control in this position so the woman can relax and enjoy the pleasure he is bringing to her body.

To get into this position, the man will stand facing a wall with the woman standing in front of him, her back to the wall. She will then jump into his arms and wrap both her arms and her legs around him. Once here, he can insert his penis into her vagina while holding onto her buttocks or underneath her knees. He can lean her back on the wall in front of him for support so that he does not have to support her entire weight in his arms. If he holds onto her underneath her knees, this will open her up so that her vagina is easily accessible. The fact that she is suspended coupled with this will make it so that there is deep penetration occurring, and this will be pleasurable for both the man and the woman. Deep penetration is great for the female orgasm because there are two places located deep within the vagina that, when stimulated, lead to a very intense orgasm for her. The penis must achieve continuous deep penetration for this to happen, and in this position, it is quite possible.

Cross-Legged Vibrating

This position allows for multiple female orgasms because it involves penetration as well as clitoral stimulation. The man will sit cross-legged, and the woman will sit on his lap, wrapping her legs around behind him. This can be done in a comfortable chair or on a bed. Once the penis is inside of the woman's vagina, he can thrust into her with his hips or lift her and down on his penis with his arms. Then, since her legs are spread wide in a cross-legged position, she can use a vibrator on her clitoris (or her hand if she doesn't have one). This position will make for possible G-Spot stimulation along with the clitoral stimulation, which can lead to a blended orgasm. It can also lead to back-to-back orgasms. This can happen if she comes clitorally, and then penetration continues, which could then lead to a G-Spot orgasm (or general vaginal orgasm). Then, there is even the possibility of her having another clitoral orgasm if she begins stimulating her clitoris again

The perch

Using a chair as a perch, the man will sit on the chair (or stool) and have the woman sit down onto him, letting him inside her. She will be facing the same way he is, both of them placing their feet on the floor. He can wrap his arms around her waist and stimulate her clitoris, or she can stimulate her clitoris while he holds her breasts. Though not a lot of visual stimulation, this position allows for a lot of touch on the male's part, giving him free rein over her body.

The plough

This position requires a bit of strength on both parties, along with a lower surface, such as a bed. In the position, the woman will lay on the edge of the bed on her stomach with her legs straight out behind her, opened slightly for the male to walk in between. As the male walks in between, he will hold her legs up, taking some of the pressure off of her. He will lift her pelvis so that he can put himself inside her while she balances on the bed on her arms or elbows. While the man is standing, holding her hips with her pelvis in the air, he will then begin thrusting (or ploughing) into her. The term comes from how the man is holding the woman, almost as if he is plowing a field or using a push mower. This requires arm and abdominal strength and stamina from the woman as well as arm strength from the male.

The Scissors

This position is a little challengingto get yourselves into, but once you do, it will be well worth the effort. To begin, the man will sit on the bed with his arms behind him, holding his weight up but leaning back. Then, he will bend one of his knees, so his leg is bent. The woman will lie down on the bed face-down and with her head at the opposite end of the bed as the man. She will spread her legs and move her body toward the man's until their bodies meet. When they meet, their bodies will look like two pairs of scissors crossed into one another. From here, the man will insert his penis into her vagina. The woman can move her body up and down on his penis, and the man can thrust into her. It may take a bit of time to develop a rhythm in this position, but when you do, you will both feel intense pleasure.

Vibrating Cowgirl

This position is an advanced spin on an ideal position, as well. You may be familiar with the cowgirl position. This position begins in the same way as that. The man is lying on his back on the bed, and the woman straddles his penis, inserting it into her. The woman will move her hips on his penis to control the depth and speed of penetration and can take control of her pleasure here. This position is great for G-Spot stimulation because of the angle at which the man's penis meets the woman's vagina. Since the penis curves upward and the G-Spot is at the front of the vagina, positions, where the man and the woman's heads are at the same end of the bed, are best for G-Spot stimulation.

What makes this position advanced is that once you are in this position, you then will bring a vibrator to the clitoris of the woman. This can be done by either the man or the woman, whichever you prefer. Because the woman is on top and sitting upright, her clitoris is exposed and thus is open and accessible by a vibrator. This will give the woman maximum pleasure as she will have both G-Spot and clitoral stimulation at the same time.

She may even be able to achieve a blended orgasm, which is a combination of two different orgasms at the same time, leading to a giant mind-blowing orgasm. If you do not have a vibrator, you can use your fingers (either the woman or the man) and stimulate the clitoris in this way. This now brings us to our next category of positions, which are *the best positions for multiple female orgasms.*

Galloping Horse

The galloping horse is an exciting, fast-paced position that allows for incredibly deep penetration. The lady has little to no control in this position, which can add to her pleasure. It requires a chair, as other seat choices will not enable the position to work correctly. To start, have the gentleman sitting down with his legs straightened and feet on the floor. Then, the lady should sit on his lap, facing him, with a leg on either side. He can then enter her while she picks her feet up off of the floor and puts them straight out behind him. He can hold her upper arms or shoulders to stop her from falling back, while also giving him leverage to thrust underneath her while she bounces on top of him. It is guaranteed to provide the ultimate deep penetration experience that will send both of you over the edge in no time.

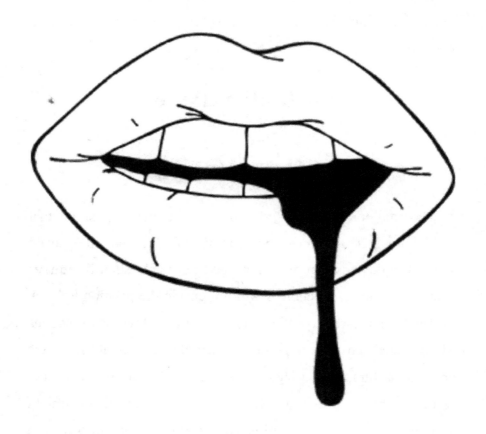

Chapter 8

Man's top 20 dominant positions

Milk the Man

This move requires some training. A woman needs to perform about 25-30 Kegel exercises a day. When she has worked her Pubococcygeus muscles to where she can isolate the inner, middle, and outer muscles, she is ready for the "milk-the-man" technique.

The man lies on his back. The woman mounts him and straddles him. She guides his penis inside of her. She then clenches her PC muscles in sequence, starting with the one that's closest to the entrance of the vagina. This will be an experience that the man has not only experienced before but didn't even know it was possible!

Multiple-Male!-Orgasms

Whenever a man has an orgasm, it's followed by a refractory period, during which he can't become erect again. Some men, this might last minutes, for others, it might last days. What most men don't know is that the release of sperm and their orgasm can be separated. When a man is about to ejaculate, press your middle firmly on the perineum (the ridge between the testicles and the anus). This will cut off the flow of semen while he has his orgasm. After the orgasm, he will find that he is immediately ready to go again.

The P-Spot

While pleasuring a man, he can be easily stimulated by massaging his prostate. This can be done externally by rubbing the perineum (the ridge between the testicles and the anus) or internally but wetting a finger with lube and slowly massaging the outer rectum. This area is rich with nerve ending and can create immense, please. Slowly insert the finger (short nails please) only a little bit, wait for the sphincter to relax before proceeding further.

The best way to massage the prostate is with the finger inside the anus, massaging what will feel like a walnut-sized sack (in the direction of the belly button). For the man with an adventurous spirit, a curved dildo can also be used to stimulate him. While this can be an incredibly gratifying experience for the man, it's important to know beforehand that he is comfortable with it.

Closed Door

This position is similar to the missionary in that both people are lying down face-to-face, and the man is on top. The difference, however, and what makes this an advanced position is that the woman will keep her legs shut the entire time tightly. The man's penis can be inserted while her legs are open, and then once it is in, she will close her legs. What this does is constrict her vagina and make the canal tighter for the man's penis. In addition to this, if she is aroused, her vagina will be engorged, and the canal will be tighter already. Because of this, the man's penis will be hugged tightly as it slides in and out of her, and this will make for extra pleasure for him.

Lap Dance

This next position is another that is best for male pleasure and the male orgasm. This position requires strength on the part of the man and the woman and is quite an athletic position, but this is why it is called an advanced sex position. Be careful when trying this one.

To get into position, the man will sit upright in a comfortable chair or on the edge of a bed with his feet planted on the floor. The woman will climb onto his lap and wrap her legs around behind the man or stick them straight out past him. Then, the man can insert his penis into the woman's vagina. From here, the woman will lean back until she is lying straight back, and her body is flat. While she does this, the man will have to hold onto her at her hips or her lower back, depending on your height variations. The man in this position will perform a combination of thrusting his hips into the woman from a seated position and pulling her onto his penis repeatedly. A high amount of upper body strength is required on the part of the man in this position. Place some pillows on the floor underneath the woman when trying this position, just in case. The woman can hold onto the man's arms for support as well here.

This position is excellent for the male's pleasure because it allows him to control the speed and depth of thrusting, and it allows for deep penetration, which will feel amazing on his penis.

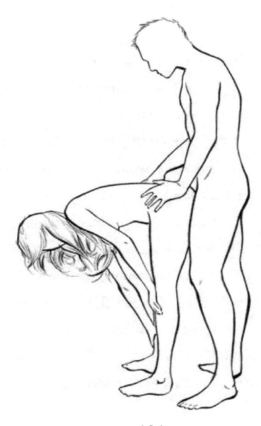

Splitting the Bamboo

This position is quintessentially Kama Sutra, and it is a great position for the male orgasm. To get into this position, the woman will lie on her back on the bed and stretch one of her legs straight out below her, lifting the other leg and resting it on the man's shoulder. The man will be on top of the woman, his hips between her legs.

In this position, the man can achieve deep penetration because of the positioning of the woman's legs, which will feel great for him. The deeper he can penetrate, the more pleasured he will be.If the woman is not flexible enough to do this position in this way, making it uncomfortable, the man can kneel instead of laying on top of her. This way, the position will still be accomplished, but it does not give the woman's leg as much of a stretch. This position is also great for the woman since the chances of G-Spot stimulation are very high.

Waterfall

The waterfall is a position in which the man has complete control. The man will begin by sitting in a chair with his feet on the floor. The woman will climb onto his lap and insert his penis into her. She can wrap her legs around his waist. Then, slowly, she will lean back until her head and arms are touching the floor (with pillows underneath). From here, the man will hold onto her hips and can move her body onto his penis at whatever speed and depth he wishes. He can also grab onto her breasts and massage her clitoris in this position if he wants. This position can be quite challenging for the woman, but the blood flow to her head will make it pleasurable for her. This position is excellent for the man since he is in control, and the tightness of the woman's vagina around his penis in this position will be hugely pleasurable for him.

Standing Suspended From Behind-Anal

This position is great for those who are experienced with anal sex as it allows for deep penetration and also requires strength from both partners. This one is a bit trickier to get into, so to begin, the man will be sitting down on the edge of the bed or in a chair, and the woman will sit on his lap, facing away from him. Then, the man will insert his penis into her anus. He will hold onto her under her knees or her buttocks, and once secure, he will stand up, still inside of her. Then, leaning his back against a wall for support, he will thrust into and out of her while holding her up. This position can be very pleasurable for both people if fitness and strength are there, which is why this is such an advanced position. This position is goodfor the male orgasm because this position and the fact that it involves anal sex will make it feel great for him. The only thing is that it requires a lot of work from the woman as well.

Manhandle-her.

This excellent position allows him to enter her from behind while having the ability to stimulate her clitoris or breasts at the same time. You can do it anywhere you'd like, as it is a standing position. You can alter it to be laying down position as well, however, by simply laying on your sides in a spooning position. It works by having the lady standing in front with her legs partially spread. Then, the gentleman comes up behind her and enters her, while using one hand to hold on (such as around her chest, while gently massaging or squeezing her breast) and using the other to stimulate her clitoris. This is an excellent position to help the lady reach orgasm, as it provides all of the stimulation necessary for her climax.

Sexy Spoons

This position is excellent for intense, slow, sensual penetration. It is another from-behind entry that is excellent for her pleasure and his. This is a relatively straight forward position that you can probably assume how it works. To start, have the lady lay on the bed on her preferred side. It is easiest if she has the top leg in front of the bottom leg. Then, have the gentleman come up behind and spoon her while penetrating her. He can use her hips as leverage to control the speed of his thrusts, or he can slowly thrust while stimulating her clitoris. She can use her free hand to massage his bum or play with her clitoris.

Pressing Position

The pressing position is one of the best and fulfilling positions you can try with your lover as it unfolds effortlessly from one embrace to a rhythm like lovemaking. This lovemaking is very sensual and can be used to connect with your partner deeply. And it is very easy to perform, and the best part is that both lovers would get to enjoy the lovemaking to the fullest.

To perform this lovemaking, lie your partner down on the bed after you must have had a series of foreplay. As she lies down on the bed, you can further go more in-depthwith the foreplay by rubbing her breast and nipples to arouse her further. Then you could go lower and play around her belly, and you approach her vagina. You could also place a kiss on her vagina, and a little clitoris stimulation would also help as you go into position for this lovemaking. Remember, your lover is already lying flat on the bed back down.

Then spread both of her legs on either side of your waist and fix yourself in-between. Then move a bit forward and place your hands at her sides and lean softly on her. Then at this position, you can go for insertion. Upon entering her vagina, go easy, it would feel a bit tight at first, but after a couple of minutes, and with the right amount of vagina fluid from arousing her well, things should go a lot smoother. The main should use his feet to apply pressure when making love in this position.

The woman could also grip her partner's thigh with her own and press it inwards to tighten her vagina to thrust his penis more thigh for more friction and pleasure, which increases the sensation for both of you. Generally, this position is great because of the body contact around the limb, and belly region as well. Moreover, the more the partners roll around together as they press their limb together, the greater the sexual charge would be.

Mare's Position

This is also another sex position from the Kama Sutra worth taking a look at as lovers. One of the advantages of this technique is that it can be done in various positions. And if the woman is those that contract during orgasm, then she could employ her vaginal muscles to squeeze her lover's penis as though she were milking the penis. This sex position is highly pleasurable, that is why I'm featuring it in this book.

To enjoy this position, as the man, you can enjoy it in two positions – either lying back down and or sitting with one hand on the bed for support. As usually, sex should always proceed after a series of foreplay. When emotions are high, and the two of you are really in the mood and want to dive into each other, then the man should go to bed. As I said earlier, you can either take a seated position of back down position.

In that position, the woman crosses her legs over yours and faces the same direction you are facing. So, her back would be at your front. In that position, before you go for congress, you can further do a little more foreplay, like kissing her back, playing with her hair, or squeezing the breast would not be a bad idea.

Then you can go for penetration as the man. On entering the vagina with your penis, you should take the lying down position at first as it helps reveals more of the penis for deeper penetration. As you penetrate, you can then sit up for more joyride. After some time enjoying this position with your partner, you feel very close to orgasm, you could take the sitting position as it helps to reduce the feeling of orgasm.

You could also help by stimulating her clitoris with your fingertips as you sit up. She could also do this herself, whichever you two lovebirds prefer would be just fine. One thing you both will enjoy again in this position is the skin contact because it is more like she is sitting on your lap. This sense alone can increase arousal to make the man have an orgasm in no time. Because you'd both feel the buttock bouncing on the laps, making those clapping sounds turning both lovers on more. This position is enjoyable, and lovers should try it out.

The Lotus

In the Kama Sutra, this is better known as the Padma.

The couple sits together in bed, facing each other.

The man pulls the woman's body close to his, grabs her ankles, raise them, and locks them behind his neck.

They make love to each other by grinding their hips together. The pleasure is in the hot rubbing sensation of the genitals.

Ensure that the genitals are amply lubricated before making love in the Lotus.

This sitting position provides lovers with the opportunity to maintain eye contact throughout sex, thus, increasing the intimacy of the act.

The Perch

The lovers start by having the man sitting on a stool with his legs spread somewhat apart.

With her back to him and leaning forward slightly to ease penetration, the woman perches herself onto the man's lap.

Using her legs, she performs up and down movements.

Meanwhile, the man reaches in front to play with his lover's breasts or to caress her clitoris.

The fan

This position is another spin-off of the commonly known and incredibly loved doggy-style position. The woman will bend forward onto a stool, table, counter, or another hard surface that is lower than she is. From this position, she will arch her back, lifting her bottom higher in the air and giving the man a much better angle for entering her. He can place his hands on her bottom or wrap them around to stimulate her clitoris (even better if this is done during anal sex). This is called the fan because the man can thrust in a circular motion, similar to a fan.

Elephant Posture

This sex position is highly recommended as it is very sensual and comes with a lot of joy attached. This position is so dominant because there are lots of body contact involved in the position. Lovers who want to connect deeply can have a fun time enjoying this position. To perform this position, very little is needed to know about from the right foreplay that would lead to this position.

To begin lovemaking in this position, start with the right foreplay that would make you get to your lovers back. Kissing her whole-body round could be a great start. Or you can combine kissing her body with a little hair play and then find your way to her back. Kiss her shoulder and bend her over until she's lying down with her stomach, thigh, breast, and feet all touching the bed. In this position, you could go for a little massaging to stimulate her even more.

Massage her back and go down a little to massage her buttocks. She rubsher around her vagina and stimulates her clitoris until she fills wet on her vagina. Then you can go for the penetration, place your hands and either side of your lover, and lean on her buttock a bit. Then like you, as you go for the penetration, pass your penis between her slightly parted legs and get into her vagina.

This sex position is very sensual as you would enjoy the feeling of her buttock around the penis, which is very pleasurable. The woman can intensify the sensation for both of you by pressing her thigh closely once the man is insider her to increase the feeling.

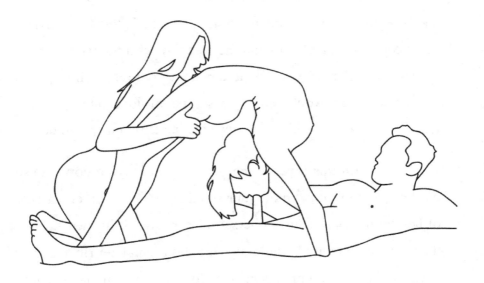

Level Feet Posture

This position is a type of Ananga Ranga way of lovemaking. This position can be a bit difficult to do and is not a position that can be enjoyed for a prolonged time. To perform this lovemaking, you need to find a way to end the foreplay with the woman back on the bed. But if you are a couple who love to have deep penetration, sex would enjoy this type of lovemaking as the position reveals the vagina in a way that penetration can go deep.

To perform this lovemaking, the woman is lying down, raise her legs, and place them on your shoulder. One leg on either side of her partner as she pushes herself closer towards his penis. Then the man supports her by holding her sides around her rib and then goes for the penetration. As he goes for the penetration, she could increase the pressure by closing her thing, which would make the penetration more pleasurable on his deep-plunging penis.

Crab Embrace Position

As lovers, if you want a sex position that you can do for a very prolonged period, then this is perfect for you. The crab and embrace position is more of a side-by-side position in the sense that you and your partner are both lying down side by side facing each other. The penetration in this position would be deep. However, the man's movement would be restricted in a way. This sex position is very sensual as you can look deep into your lover's eyes as you make love and use your hands to caress each other. You both could even have a deep sensual kiss in-between the sex.

To perform this inviting and warm sex position, the man would lie right next to the woman and places one of his legs in-between her legs. In this lying position, he then goes for the penetration. And like I said earlier, the penetration movement wouldn't be much, so done expect too much movement. This position is also great, especially when you and your lover have been having sex for a prolonged time, and you are both tired but still passionate about having sex.

When the sex is going on in this position, you can add loving caresses to the mix. Use your free hand to caress each other's face, torso, arms, thighs, and buttocks. Again, the leg position is also important in this sex position, so make sure you put your uppermost leg over his body and rest your knee back to his hip.

Rainbow Arch Position

It is never a bad idea to try something new, and this sex position is going to be something new in your archive. This sex position is somewhat tricky, but when you get a hold of the idea of the position, it will come in a lot easier. This sex position is a side by side sec position, and the posture has an unusual angle for penetration, which has a very sensational feeling attached.

To perform this sex position with your lover, you and your lover are to lie down flat on the bed. As the woman lies down, she is to raise one of her legs, sure that the man can fix himself in-between her opened legs. The man should set himself, in-between her legs in such a way that his face goes to the back of the woman while his legs come to her front. Then as he goes for the penetration, he holds her shoulder to make the movement easier. She can keephis leg for support, so she doesn't move too much while the man applies more pressure for the lovemaking.

Driving the Peg Home

This is a standing posture sex position. It might involve some strength from the man's side, but it is definitely worth the power. Strength is needed in the sense that the man would need to lift the woman for the penetration. So, for lovers to enjoy this sex position, the man needs to be strong so that he can thrust his penis satisfactorily while bearing the weight of his partner. However, great care is needed because his member is very vulnerable to damage in this position, so he should take great care when making love with this position.

To perform this position. The man should lift the woman and support her up by holding her buttocks. Then she is to thrust her legs at either side of her lover but to hold on to her lover's waist tightly while she holds his shoulder. She is also to keep her back straight as she leans against the wall.

Kneeling Fox

The kneeling fox is a spin-off of the classic doggy-style. This position allows him to penetrate her deeply while going as fast or as slow as he wants. She can also grind her hips back to meet his thrusts and further deepen the penetration. It works by having the gentleman sitting on the bed on his knees. Then, the lady squats on all fours, then sits back on his lap. He can then hold her hips as leverage, while she grinds her hips backward to meet his thrusts. This will help increase the level of penetration and help her gain control overwhere he is stimulating her.

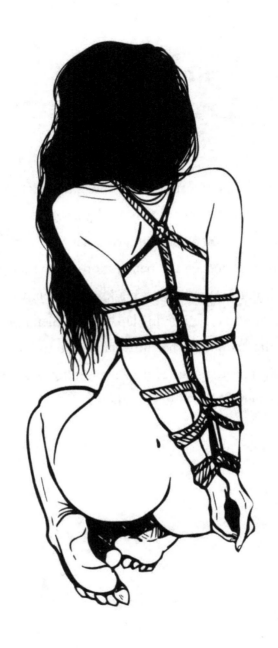

Chapter 9

The top 8 sitting positions

The Tortoise

The other name for this position in the Kama Sutra is the Kaurma. The couple begins by sitting together in bed, facing each other. The man raises his feet and caresses the woman's nipples with his toes. The woman does the same, resting her feet on her man's chest. They hold each other's hands, and together, they develop a slow and sensual rhythm with their hips.

The Swing

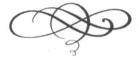

This sitting sex position is called the Dolita in the Kama Sutra.

The lovers sit face to face in bed.

They draw their bodies close to each other so that the woman's breasts are pressed tightly against her lover's chest.

The couple wraps their legs around each other's bodies and locks their heels about each other's waist.

Both lean their bodies backward while holding on to each other's wrists.

With the man's penis buried deep inside the woman, the lovers swing gently to and fro.

The Peacock

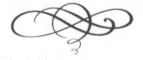

The sacred name of this sitting sex position is the Mayura.

The woman sits on the bed and raises one leg so that it is pointing skyward.

She uses her hands to steady the leg as she offers her sacred flower to her lover.

Note: For this position, the woman needs to be flexible enough.

The Knot of Flame

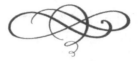

In the ancient texts, this is also known as the Kirti bandha.

The man and the woman sit up straight on the bed with their legs in front of them.

Next, the man holds onto his partner's waist.

He then pulls her body close to his.

They both plunge into each other with hardcore thrusts.

The Frog

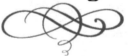

The lovers start with the man seated in the corner of the bed and with his feet planted firmly on the floor.

The woman settles herself down on his penis by squatting with her feet planted on the bed.

Her back should be against her lover. This way, she resembles a frog about to jump.

The woman then bounces up and down her lover while holding onto his thighs.

Meanwhile, the man supports her by placing his hands beneath her bottom to give her a bit of a lift.

If the woman is strong enough to do the up and down movements on her own, the man may use his hands to reach in front and massage her breasts or tickle her love button.

The Kneel

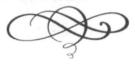

This is more of a kneeling sex position than a sitting one, but it's delightful because it provides the lovers with the opportunity to wrap their arms around each other and engage in a romantic lip-lock while doing the deed.

The man and the woman both assume a kneeling position in bed while facing each other.

The woman straddles her man. He then penetrates her, and while he does, she envelops his neck in her arms.

The man embraces his lover. Using his knees, he moves slowly up and down.

The Boat

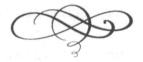

The couple starts by having the man lay down on a supine position.

The woman then settles herself down on him.

Then, the man sits up gradually while pulling his knees up. This way, he and his lover are now sitting face to face.

The woman's legs should be on either side of the man's torso.

Likewise, the man's legs should be on either side of her torso.

The man is to slide his arms over the woman's calves and under her knees.

Meanwhile, the woman is to slide her hands under the man's knees and then around her thighs. This way, she would be able to hold her lover's hands in hers while they are making love.

The Sacred Chair

The man settles himself comfortably on a stool with his feet together.

Facing him, the woman sits down on his lap with her legs on either side of his body.

She leans forward and clings to her lover.

Her feet should be firmly planted in the ground so that she can bounce herself up and down with ease.

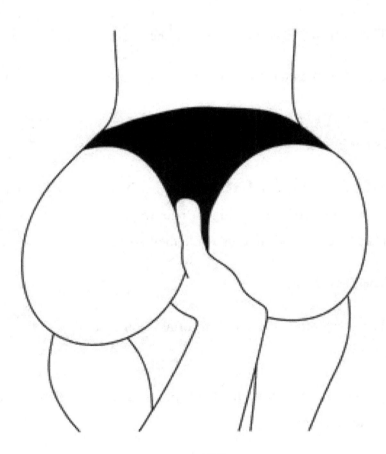

Chapter 10

Masturbation for women

For many women, masturbation is more than a means of gratifying oneself when they are single. It's their way of learning the complexities of their bodies, of teaching themselves how to work all the different parts of their body and bring themselves to orgasm.

Everyone woman is different. The stimulations and time frames can vary greatly, and if left to their partner to figure out, it could take exponentially longer for them to learn what it takes to have an orgasm. Just as we are accountable for our happiness, we are also accountable for how well we know our bodies.

We cannot expect our partners to understand what we desire when we haven't spent much time trying to figure it out, or as is often the case, we are too timid to give voice to what we want or need in the bedroom.

The Kama Sutra barely mentions masturbation. If anything, there's an implication that men shouldn't do it. And yet, for a lot of the positions proposed in the book, masturbation would be an excellent tool for both the man and the woman to prepare themselves for lovemaking sessions that will require endurance and a clear understanding ofhow each person prefers to be stimulated. After all, who knows more than you on how to get you off?

As odd as it may sound, masturbation can also fall into a routine. There are small things that can be done to spice up the one-person show: men who always favor their left, or right hand might enjoy switching things up, and using the other sideand trying a different lotion can awaken different nerve fibers.

Thanks to the Internet, there is a never-ending supply of pornographic material to feed one's masturbation sessions. It's as easy as typing in a few keywords, and a library of videos matching your specifications will pop up. Often, old favorites will be revisited, and being adventurous is nothing more than finding a new video to feed one's imagination.

This method is incredibly popular because it works. Still, for many, it would be a revelation to forego porn for a session and allow their imagination to come up with its scenario. At first, the mind might conjure up images that were embedded by the videos. Still, if one is committed to exploring new desires within themselves, they'll push past ideas and scenarios that have already been played out in their mind many times.

Try to imagine a new position, a new place, or perhaps a new role that you've never thought about before. By challenging yourself, you will be much more likely to challenge your partner the next time you make love.

For some, the challenge with masturbation is their guilt. Religion, inhibitions, or conservative views about sex can stifle a person's willingness to masturbate. Should the desire build to an irresistible point, the act becomes so rushed and immediately followed by shame. This can rob the person an incredible tool forlearning their likes and dislikes.

On the more practical side of things, masturbation can be used as practice for a man's endurance. For those who reach climax quickly, masturbating can be a great time to master, delaying the climax. This can feel a bit torturous at first, but for the frustration, this can create, it makes up for it when one applies their skills during lovemaking.

This is especially true when trying new positions. As both partners try to find angles, positions, and rhythms for each technique, it's useful if the man manages to stay erect. Reaching one's climax or losing their arrival, prematurely can take all the fun out of practicing new positions.

For many men, the idea of showing their partner how they masturbate is too awkward to consider. And yet, the expectation for a woman to effectively provide handjobs or help keep a man aroused is quite common. Even if a woman has experience from previous relationships, every man's sensitivity is different. And the man has the most to gain by showing his partner the strokes, pace, and any other tricks he uses to get himself to climax.

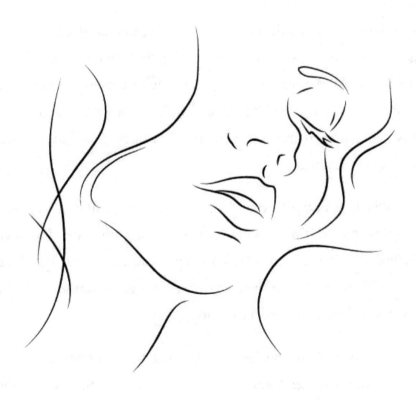

Chapter 11

Anal sex

Anal sex is something that not everyone has had experience with. It has the potential to provide you and your partner with very great pleasure if you know how to safely and comfortably engage in this type of sex. In this chapter, I will explain how you can safely have anal sex and how you can begin to use it to your advantage to experience pleasure like never before.

Lubricate

Unlike the vagina, the anus does not lubricate itself naturally. Therefore, you have to use a lubricant. Many on the market are warming, as well as some that are intended to help relax the muscles and make anal a more enjoyable experience for the lady. You should opt for a water-based lubricant of your choice. The key to anal sex is lubrication! You will need to make sure that both the penis (or dildo) and the anus are well-lubricated for anal sex to be pleasurable for everyone involved. The anus doesn't lubricate itself asthe vagina does, so you have to make sure you do it yourselves before having anal sex.

Relax

As the lady, you want to make sure you relax your muscles and take deep breaths. Go slow and take care not to tense up out of fear. To help reduce tensing up due to fear, make sure you follow the next step carefully.

Start Small

Especially if you are brand new to anal, as, in an anal virgin, you will want to start very small, using plenty of lube, and a littletoy or his pinky finger, he can gently work his way into your bum and help you relax the muscles. He should move slowly and at your discretion, to ensure you are prepared for every step.

Go Slow

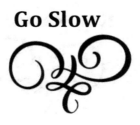

Aside from working your way up slowly, all movements should be slow as well. Once you're used to it and have more confidence in the experience, you can start going faster. But every single anal experience should beginwith slow movements and shallow penetration. From there, he can choose how deep and quick he will go, based on how she feels.

Communicate

This is the one time you especially want to communicate well during sex. The lady should always be telling the gentleman if what he is doing is okay, and he should not be doing anything she doesn't like or that hurts her. You can even enforce a safe word that means you stop completely if one party is not enjoying themselves or is hurt by it.

Relaxation

The next point to keep in mind is relaxation. The anus will open gradually as you start to play around and inside of it a little bit. As you slide something into it, it will respond by opening up and relaxing, but this may take a few minutes. Having aperson be relaxed and comfortable is very important. Remember to let it do its thing, and just slowly enjoy the process without rushing it. If the person is too nervous, it will take longer for their anus to relax.

Removal

The next thing to note is that if you are going to remove something like a toy or a penis from the anus, it is important to make sure the person is relaxed and lubricated (as stated above). More importantly, they must be expecting the removal of whatever was inserted into their anus to happen. If you try to remove it without the person expecting it quickly, their body will reflexively tense the anus, and it will lead to a painful experience, possibly for both people if it was a penis inserted.

Remembering these three points will help you to have a positive and enjoyable anal sex experience for your first time. There are a few more things to note to ensure that you have safe anal sex. These points are related to hygiene and sex toys and will likely become more relevant when you are more experienced with anal sex.

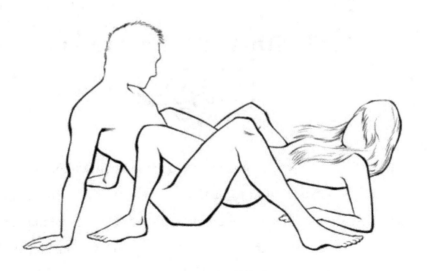

Kama Sutra Positions for Anal Sex

The following positions are great for people who are new to anal sex and would like to try some of the more straightforwardpositions to get used to the feeling of anal sex. These positions are straight from the Kama Sutra, or slight variations of Kama Sutra positions to make them optimized for anal sex.

Oral with Anal Stimulation

This first position is not involving anal penetration with a penis but is an excellent introduction to anal play. This position is done when a woman is giving a man oral sex. The man stands up, and the woman is on her knees in front of him, giving him oral sex. She will then reach around behind the man's buttocks and stimulate his anus with her finger. She can move her finger around the outside of his anus, stimulating the sensitive skin there, which will make him feel immense amounts of pleasure. Giving oral sex and stimulating his anus at the same time will make it virtually impossible for him not to orgasm very quickly.

The Curled Angel

This is a Kama Sutra position that is written as a position to be performed with vaginal sex, but it can also be done as an anal sex position. This position involves the man and woman lying down on their sides, the man behind the woman. Both of them are facing the same direction, so the curve of their hips places the man's penis at the perfect point for anal penetration. In this position, the man and woman can grind their hips into each other, and it is a team effort in terms of control.

The Clip

In this position, the man lies back on the bed with his knees bent and his feet planted on the bed. The woman straddles the man and inserts his penis into her anus. In this position, she can lean forward onto the man's bent knees for support, and she can control the depth and speed of penetration. The man can hold onto the woman's buttocks and guide her movements as well.

The Snake

This position is a good one to try when you have a little bit of experience with anal sex but are not ready to try anything too extreme just yet. The person receiving anal penetration in this position takes a passive role and can just focus on relaxing and enjoying the pleasure rather than having to contort into some type of acrobatic formation.

To begin, the woman will lie face down on the bed, and her partner will lie on top of her, supporting himself with his arms.

From here, the woman will arch her back a bit to make her pleasure zones as accessible as possible for penetration. Now, the man will slowly slide his penis into her anus. Here, the woman can enjoy the pleasure ride her partner takes her on, without having to do anything herself. She can enjoy these moments where the focus is all on her!

Pegging

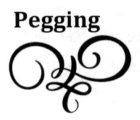

There is another type of anal sex that can be had, which involves sex toys. It is quite common that a woman will penetrate her male partner anally while wearing a strap-on. This practice is called Pegging. Now that you know a little more about sex toys and anal sex, and how to ensure you are combining these two in a safe and sanitary way, you are ready to try Pegging. This can be done either by using a dildo placed in a strap-on that a woman is wearing or by using a double-ended dildo. Using a double-ended dildo will allow the woman to be pleasured at the same time as she is penetrating the man, as she will also be penetrated either vaginally or anally with the other end of the dildo. This type of dildo looks like any other, except that it has two identical ends.

Now that you are aware of the possibility of this type of practice, you can understand how any of these anal sex positions can be performed by either the man penetrating the woman anally with his penis or by the woman penetrating her partner anally using a dildo.

For men, anal sex is extremely pleasurable since their prostate is stimulated through anal penetration. The prostate is what has been referred to as the "male G-Spot."

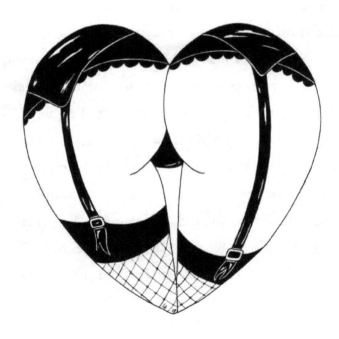

Chapter 12

Super orgasm

For many people, when it comes to lovemaking, the orgasm isn't the cherry on top. It's the entire sundae. They treat foreplay and intercourse as if there were playing poker, and if they play their cards right, they win the pot and cash those chips in for a mind-blowing, body quivering orgasm.

What if they don't climax? Well, then they treat the whole experience as though they won the pot only to discover the chips can't be cashed in. They're stuck with two handfuls of cheapplastic. Everyone can agree that orgasms feel amazing. It's a sure sign that all the elements in lovemaking came together correctly to give that partner a moment of ecstasy.

As great as they are, it's a huge mistake to make that the goal of lovemaking, especially when practicing the Kama Sutra. When practicing the techniques, the experience shouldn't be a judge on whether or not one or both partners experienced orgasms. In fact, they shouldn't even be basing it on how close they came to climaxing. Orgasms can be very elusive, especially for women.

Sometimes it might take more time than they have. Sometimes thinking about it makes it difficult actually to have it. Sometimes, it doesn't happen because it just didn't happen.

Male Orgasm Basics

The male orgasm is something that most people have witnessed or seen if they have ever watched any sort of porn or heard about it in the media. The male orgasm is made out to be extremely simple and easy to achieve, but in this section, we are going to examine it in more detail and break it down into more specific parts.

To start, are you aware that there are different types of male orgasms? If you are a male, you are likely aware of this, but if you are a female, you may not be. The term *male orgasm* includes any and every type of orgasm that involves the male's genitals.

Orgasm and Ejaculation

Ejaculation and orgasm for males are two distinct events, even though they most often happen at the same time. This fact makes them often misunderstood, as many think that ejaculation is a sign of orgasm. If orgasm occurs and ejaculation occurs at the same time, this is called an **ejaculatory orgasm.**

There is another type of orgasm, one that happens when ejaculation does not. As you likely guessed, this type is called a **non-ejaculatory orgasm.** This is sometimes called a *dry orgasm* as well, and this type is also very normal. A man can achieve orgasm without ejaculation, and this still counts as an orgasm.

How to Stimulate the Prostate to Achieve Orgasm

Once you have found the prostate, you can begin to massage this area and let the sensations build gently. Keep going like this and find out what type of movements or pressure feels best. As you continue to stimulate it, let the pleasure makeuntil the point of orgasm. When you are comfortable with this spot, try having your partner encourage it for you. Having someone else's hands touch it for you will feel different than your own, and with your free hand, you can turn yourself and your partner on in other ways.

The prostate is sometimes referred to as the male G-Spot. It has many similar properties to the female G-Spot, such as the way that you can find it and how it needs t to be stimulated to reach orgasm. We will learn about the female orgasm in the following section.

Female Orgasm Basics

To make a woman orgasm, you will need to know and understand the female body, including all of the places where, when stimulated, a woman will feel pleasure and maybe even orgasm. Whether you are a female yourself or you are a male with a female partner, both sexes can benefit from learning more about the female body.

How to Stimulate the Clitoris to Achieve Orgasm

Once you have found the clitoris, you will then be able to stimulate it to achieve orgasm. Begin by gently placing two fingers on it and putting a bit of pressure. Rub it by moving your fingers in small circles-making sure to be gentle. Continue to do this, and she should begin to get more aroused the more you do this. By rubbing the clitoris, you will be able to stimulate the entire clitoris, even the part of it that you cannot see, and this will cause the woman to start to become wet in her vaginal area for her body to prepare for sex.

How to Stimulate the G-Spot to Achieve Orgasm

To give a woman pleasure by stimulating her G-Spot, you will need to press on it over and over again until she reaches orgasm. The G-Spot needs to receive continued and consistent stimulation for the pleasure to build enough for her to reach orgasm. This can be done using your fingers, a penis, or sex toys of a variety of sorts.

Since a woman can have two different types of orgasms, one from stimulating the clitoris and a different one from penetration or hitting the G-spot, this could be why a woman can reach orgasm during oral sex, or by having her clitoris stimulated, but has trouble reaching the same level of pleasure during penetrative sex. In many positions, the G-spot is not stimulated by the man's penis, and this can result in the woman having some amount of pleasure, but not enough to reach orgasm. For a great experience as a couple, knowing what makes the woman feel great is paramount.

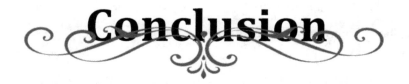

Conclusion

The Kama Sutra is the epitome of an intimate sexual relationship. This book has covered all of the basics, especially about how the Kama Sutra is about more than just sex. It is about the connection with your partner on an emotional and spiritual level. This book is written to teach a novice about how to set the mood, and how to hold your partner, with a few positions to try out.

The Kama Sutra is about loving your partner and showing them by exploring every inch of their body. It is not about being considered a "sex god," but about being an attentive lover.

Remember, sex is an incredibly important part of romantic relationships. There are a ton of health benefits related to having sex regularly, including improved immunity, increased heart health, lower blood pressure, pain relief, decreased stress and improved sleep, better libido, and so much more. After reading this book, I hope you were able to gain a fantastic understanding of past and current sexual activities along with a variety of different ways to spice up your own sex life and enjoy yourself and your lover on a more intimate and sensual level. Sex can be as intimate or as shallow as you make it; however, meaningful and passionate sex is almost always preferred. With this book, you should be able to understand the initial purpose of the Kama Sutra and the principles that surrounded it.

One of the most significant issues in today's relationships is that people aren't exploring each other's bodies the way they used to. With this book, I hope you can enter the bedroom with confidence to please your loved one and the willingness to do whatever it takes; and I hope they feel the same way. The Kama Sutra was right when it spoke of finding someone compatible with you anatomically and attitude-wise. Someone who has a high sex drive isn't going to mesh well with someone who has a low sex drive. You may be able to make it work on an emotional level, but on a physical and sexual level, your relationship may fall short.

Granted, sex isn't everything in a relationship, but it means more to some people in a relationship than it does to others, so choose your lover wisely. This book should have also shown you different ways in which women may have seen you in the past and the future; the same goes for women and how men view them. In modern times, we don't care muchaboutthe way people see us, but in ancient times, your reputation was everything. This book can be an eye-opener to how some of your current behaviors may have been seen in ancient times – whether that affects you or not is your own accord.

Aside from many asinine doings involved in recipes, spells, and charms, there was also a lot of educational and exciting information on aphrodisiac foods and which ones work the best. Some people might not even realize the large numberof foods that can be arousing to specificindividuals. We all have thethings that arouse us – scribble that in on the aphrodisiac section.

It is very easy to slip into a life of routine, which isn't necessarily a bad thing unless it has to do with your sex life and learning. Two things you should never stop doing: learning and experimenting in the bedroom. Take the knowledge you have received from this book as either a grain of salt or as your new sexual bible. I hope you enjoyed it!

Because it's tough to find a partner who fulfills every desire of yours, and nothing could be able to replace this type of loss. So, to keep on reading this passage if you have some importance of your partner and want to cope with a problem like premature ejaculation and not satisfying your partner in bed.

The connection of the bodies should not end with orgasm but should continue long after both are replete. A man and woman should come together in mind, body, and spirit. Such is the essence of the Kama Sutra; such is the Art of Love.

CPSIA information can be obtained
at www.ICGtesting.com
Printed in the USA
LVHW010214211120
672009LV00006B/511